DEALING

WITH

CLIMATE CHANGE &

STRESS

By Captain Paul Watson

Nothing in life is to be feared, it is only to be understood. Now is the time to understand more, so that we may fear less.
- *Marie Curie*

1

THE SITUATION

The most significant survival threat we face today is climate change.

One of the consequences of climate change is the emergence of new viruses.

We are now officially in a global pandemic. However, more significantly, we have been under threat from Climate Change for decades.

This is however a serious highly contagious virus and all proper precautions must be taken.

Most importantly we need to practice social distancing. No crowds, no handshakes, hugs or meetings.

We need to avoid contact with other people as much as possible and to wash our hands and disinfect surfaces.

In short, we need to be mindful.

Most importantly we must not stress about this situation. Worry will not solve the problem and may contribute to the weakening of our immune systems. Stress suppresses the immune system and only serves to make the body more vulnerable.

For this reason. I have prepared this little booklet on dealing with stress in general and applying this advice, especially to alleviating stress over the Covid-19 virus and climate change.

I have no intention of downplaying the seriousness of the virus or the seriousness overall of climate change.

The Covid-19 virus is very dangerous and especially so to older people and to people who are immune deficient or have respiratory issues, heart issues, high blood pressure or diabetes.

People are sick. People will get sick. People have died and more people will die. These are facts. I am at myself at 69 in the high-risk category.

Normal hygienic practices can help to prevent the spread of the virus and proper care should be obtained if infected.

Do people have existing medical issues or if elderly, it is a serious concern.

However, there is no point in stressing about becoming sick.

Can Covid-19 kill you? Yes, that is a real concern.

Will Covid-19 kill you? Most likely not.

Will being stressed about these facts weaken your immune system? The answer is most likely?

And finally, will being stressed about the situation help you to deal with the situation. The answer is absolutely not. It will most likely make you less able to deal with the disease.

For this reason, I believe that the advice on stress that I have been giving to my crews for four decades now can be helpful for anyone afflicted with worry and stress.

Sea Shepherd is a global operation and we have hundreds of volunteers from dozens of nations serving on our 12 ships based in areas around the planet.

The work that we do in opposing criminal poaching operations and weathering conditions in hostile and remote environments   is dangerous and can be considered to be very stressful.

Over the years I have had to council many crewmembers during these difficult situations ranging from savage storms and dangerous ice conditions to being physically assaulted by poachers.

On ships I have found that fear and worry can be contagious and a formidable obstacle to the successful completions of our missions.

In dealing with any mission the most important consideration is that we prepare for fear, worry and stress.

Fear, worry and stress are attitudes and although there can be physical and emotional damage caused by fear, worry and stress, the approach to dealing with stress can alleviate and/or remove the physical and emotional consequences.

There are some people who insist that we have no control over suffering stress. The fact is that it is an emotional response and we can indeed dismiss it or control it.

The exception is depression and people who suffer from acute anxiety and panic attacks, but I don't believe it is true for the average person. We can deal with stress in our own lives

either completely or at least by
diminishing it.

WHO AM I TO SPEAK ABOUT STRESS?

I have been leading campaigns as a ship's captain and expedition leader since 1974 and I have often been asked how I deal with stress considering the nature of my work and the numerous death threats and legal challenges, plus the many dangerous campaigns that we undertake.

The answer to this is simple. I don't deal with stress, because I do not suffer from stress. This may seem like a bold statement, perhaps even pretentious but it is accurate and it is the reason that I have successfully led hundreds of campaigns and voyages without having a single member killed or injured over a span of four decades.

9

These campaigns include ten voyages to Antarctica and the Southern Ocean, ten campaigns to oppose the slaughter of seals off Newfoundland and Labrador, a campaign to hunt down elephant poachers in East Africa, a landing in Soviet Siberia and a confrontation with the Soviet Navy plus confrontations with the Norwegian, Danish, Portuguese and Ecuadorian navies and numerous confrontations with poachers around the world. We have been fired on, depth charged, attacked with Molotov cocktails, rammed, attacked by mobs and we have had our ships sabotaged and sunk.

The challenge was not for myself. I dealt with my fears many years ago after a very near-death experience that significantly changed my life and the way I responded to danger and stress.

I am not a doctor. I am simply a sea captain with decades of experience in "stressful" situations. This is my advice.

IT IS WHAT IT IS

It is what it is. Whatever the issue, whatever the threat, whatever the circumstances it simply is what it is. Stressing will not change the situation. All problems can be dealt with through action and determination, win or lose.

Back in the Spring of 1973 when I was twenty-two years old, I learned a very valuable lesson from a very wise man.

It was in the small South Dakota village of Wounded Knee on the Lakota Oglala Pine Ridge reservation.

I was a medic working with the American Indian Movement during the militant occupation of the town in retaliation for the murder of Raymond Yellow Thunder, a member of the

Oglala people. It was a demand for justice, not just for this one murder but for many and the years of subjugation and abuse suffered by indigenous people throughout North America.

The U.S. government responded to the occupation with a very heavy hand. The U.S. Marshalls, the F.B.I. and the military. On March 3rd, Air Force F-4 Phantom Jets flew intimidatingly low over the village. The 82nd Airborne Division sent armored Personal Carriers.

The Nixon government gave orders to shoot to kill and every night I could see the tracer bullets coming in from all sides. One night while walking down the hill from the Catholic church, a bullet whistled by my ear. I had felt somewhat safe in the dark because I was unaware that the snipers had star-scopes that could see us. When the shot narrowly missed me, it occurred to me that a bullet could hit me if I was walking or crawling.

Forty-six people were hit and two men Frank Clearwater and Buddy Lamont were killed.

I realized that with such odds against us and the cow boyish attitude of the Federal agents, that we really did not stand a chance. We could not win this thing.

I asked AIM leader Russell Means about this. "Why were we continuing to hold this ground if we could not win? The odds against us were overwhelming. Should we not just surrender?"

He smiled and said, "We're not concerned about the odds against us and we are not concerned about winning or losing. We are here because this is the right place to be, the right time to be here and the right thing to do."

I was impressed and it left a lasting impression ever since. With every confrontation situation I have never been concerned about the odds against us or thoughts about winning or losing.

In August 1981, I landed with two crew on the beach in Soviet Siberia where two armed Soviet soldiers were patrolling. Our objective was to document evidence of illegal whaling operations and we did so. The soldiers just assumed that we had to be Soviet scientists. No one had invaded the Soviet Union since World War II.

For forty minutes we filmed everything. We had our evidence and we calmly walked back to our small inflatable boat.

As Eric Schwartz and Bob Osborn got into the boat I pushed it off the beach and was preparing to jump aboard when one of the Soviet soldiers approached and curtly barked, "Sto eta?" as he pointed at our boat. (What is that?)

I quickly replied, "eta Zodiac." He quickly pointed at the outboard motor and said "eta Mercury."

I did not hesitate, I turned my back and jumped into the boat quietly asking my two crew to tell me what the soldier was doing.

"He's taking down his rifle."

Quickly I told my crew to smile and wave at him. They did so. Confused he put down his rifle and began running towards the town as he sped back to our ship the *Sea Shepherd II* drifting about a mile offshore.

With the evidence in hand we headed south along the coast of Siberia and about an hour later two helicopter gunships began to buzz us and to fire flares across our bow.

I ignored them.

A half hour later a huge Soviet frigate sped towards us, came alongside us and began to signal us to stop. I refused.

At this point some of my crew began to freak out, demanding that I stop and obey the Soviet captain. I had them escorted off the bridge and locked them out.

The captain of the frigate called on the VHF radio. "Stop your ship and prepare to be boarded by the Soviet Union."

I quickly replied, "We don't have room for the Soviet Union."

We continued on heading towards international waters. He threatened to shoot. I ignored him and kept going.

We reached the boundary, crossed the line and the pursuit ended.

Later confronted by some angry crew, I told them that there was no other option. We needed to get our evidence out and surrendering would mean the failure of the mission and most likely our arrest and detainment for an unspecified amount of time. I told them that I counted on the fact that the Soviet system did not encourage individual initiative and neither the soldiers or the frigate captain did not want to make a move without absolute authority to do so.

The odds were against us yet we won the day and the mission was a success.

The situation was what it was and I had refused to entertain the idea of surrendering. We were all in and the consequences would be what they would do. I decided without hesitation to focus on the success of the mission.

So how does this relate to the presently occurring pandemic or to climate change?

Everyone needs to accept that this pandemic is real and it is a threat. It will have a serious impact on society, materially, socially and economically.

The pandemic however is a mild threat compared to the devastation that climate change will bring.

But it is what it is. These things can't be wished away and all the stressing, worrying and fear in the world will not change the situation.

A pandemic needs to be dealt with as positively and as urgently as possible. Precautions need to be implemented to prevent infection and to not spread infection. We need to think rationally and we must be mindful of the feelings and the movements of other people. We need to politely urge people to not have physical contact and to avoid situations where there is a danger of transmission of the virus.

If infected, we need to understand the symptoms.

Coronavirus disease (COVID-19) is characterized by mild symptoms including a runny nose, sore throat, cough, and fever. Illness can be more severe for some people and can lead to pneumonia or breathing difficulties.

More rarely, the disease can be fatal. Older people, and people with other medical conditions (such as asthma, diabetes, or heart disease), may be more vulnerable to becoming severely ill.

If infected, seek help, but stressing about the situation will not make things any better.

Climate change however forces us to face a far more serious threat. Again, it is what it is and we need to stand tall and to face the consequences of what our societies have wrought. Stressing about it will change nothing. Acceptance followed by passionate activism plus courage and imagination will find a solution or not, and if not, we can only do what we can do but we should never surrender. There are no inevitabilities. Life is resilient and strong. Removing stress increases your chances of survival.

IT'S ALWAYS SOMETHING

"It's always something."

I say this all the time to my crews whenever a problem arises. "It's always something and if it's not something, it's something else, but it is always something."

This means that life comes with obstacles, challenges and problems. Problems should not be unexpected. They are inevitable. All problems can be dealt with by dealing with them, delegating someone else to deal with them, or ignoring them. One thing for sure, on a ship, it is definitely always something.

And this is the case for anything in society. We should always have expectations that something can go wrong and that an accident can happen. There is always the possibility that things will not go as planned and therefore the unexpected should always be expected.

I am never surprised when things go wrong and if I'm not surprised there is no reason for disappointment.

The way to deal with this is to be prepared to change your plans or to redirect without hesitation.

In 1993 I was on my way to the Danish Faroe Islands to intervene against the killing of pilot whales and dolphins with my ship the *Cleveland Amory* when we suffered a crankcase explosion in one of the two main engines. This severely reduced our speed and our ability, rendering pointless our continuation across the North Atlantic.

The crew were disappointed but I simply told them there would be a change of plans. We were on the Grand Banks of Newfoundland and that meant there was a conservation issue that we could address.

Canada had called a moratorium on cod fishing on the Banks but just outside on the tail of the Grand Banks, Spanish and Cuban trawlers were taking cod. Without hesitation we intervened and created an international incident by blocking the trawlers, an action that resulted in my arrest by the Canadian government.

I saw it as an excellent opportunity to focus attention on the diminishment of cod fish and the collapse of the fisheries.

Canada charged me with three counts of criminal mischief although I did not injure anyone nor did I damage any property.

During the trial, the St. John's Evening Telegram reported that "everyone seemed to be very stressed out (prosecutor, judge, layers, media) except the accused who appeared to be having a good time."

After a two-week trial I was acquitted but during that time I did not see any advantage in stressing about the situation. My attitude was that the situation was what it was and there was nothing to be achieved by stressing or worrying about the possible consequences.

Problems, disappointments, and unexpected issues are a constant part of life. We just simply need to accept this and not to stress about it.

As Richard Carlson once famously said, "Don't sweat the small stuff and it's all small stuff."

STAY CALM

There really is nothing worth getting upset about. You spill some red wine on the white carpet. It happened, so getting all stressed about it will not clean the carpet.

Once when I lost my wallet and car keys I had to admit it was damn inconvenient but I was not stressed about it. I made the calls to replace the credit cards, the driver's license and the keys and that was the end of it.

These are minor things but staying calm can save your life. Once when my regulator jammed at 30 meters, I calmly signaled my partner to indicate my situation. Fretting about it will not recover the object. Panicking will not save your life. Anger emanates from stress. Without stress there can be no anger. Without stress there is no panic.

In every confrontation situation that I have been in I have stayed calm because staying calm allows me to focus and being focused is what can keep us alive in a dangerous situation.

Many years ago, I was washing my hands in a Seattle bus station men's room when three guys approached me from behind and demanded my money. One had a knife.

I turned and smiled and said, "I'm sorry I'm from Canada and we really don't do this shit there." And I walked past them. They did not stop me leaving.

People simply don't know how to deal with an unexpected reaction.

Many people are put off guard if you remain calm and focused.

In the midst of a pandemic staying focused and mindful can save your life. You need to be conscientious about washing your hands, wearing gloves, not shaking hands and keeping your distance.

If you do become infected, again keep calm. Monitor your symptoms and if it looks like it may be severe, contact a doctor and request instructions if you should have medical attention, where and when.

A panicked person can only endanger themselves and others.

Being calm means dealing with situations rationally and mindfully.

In some situations, in the past while on the bridge, some crew have panicked, and in a few cases, became hysterical and irrational.

As an example, while trapped in thick ice off the coast of Antarctica in 2002, it looked like there was no way out and we were 2,330 miles from Australia. I told the crew to relax and reminded them that Ernest Shackleton had his ship totally crushed in worst conditions and his crew all survived. They survived by not panicking and keeping their minds focused on dealing with problems rationally.

I began to push through the ice putting pressure on the hull just aft of the bow. We had a cameraman down there filming as the ice ground against the hull and pushed. We could see the steel hull plates buckling under the pressure.

The cameraman fled, saying he had not signed up for this. I said to the other three crew with me that there really was no problem. If the hull was breached, the water would pour into the watertight compartment we were in and would rise only to the level of the water outside and we could easily climb out and if need be we could patch the hole later.

Later I asked the cameraman why he fled? He replied that his fear was that the ship would sink if the hull was breached. I told him that the situation was under control but if the ship did sink 2300 miles from Australia, we were all in the same boat and we would deploy the lifeboats and issue a mayday.

He said again, "I did not sign up for this."

"What did you sign up for?" I asked. You signed onboard a ship going to the Southern Ocean through ice and storms. You did indeed absolutely sign onto this. If you wanted a risk-free pleasure trip you should have stayed at home. But think about it, look on the positive side. We are having an exciting and adventurous voyage. It does not come risk free."

"But we could die down here."

"That is quite possible," I replied. "But you could have died in a car accident back home crossing the street. But it sure as hell would not have been this exciting now, would it?"

"Keep calm and enjoy the campaign. Chances are you will not die but if you do, well we will all die someday, somehow. The point is to enjoy your life and your experiences without getting all stressed about it."

FEAR

One of my favorite quotes is by
Franklin D. Roosevelt when he said,
"The only thing we have to fear is
fear itself."

It is fear that cripples us, disables us
and obstructs us.

The thing that people fear most is
death.

As a child I almost died three times.
Twice I almost drowned and the third
time when I was afflicted with scarlet
fever.

I survived without a fear of water. In
fact, I have embraced water all my
life from swimming to scuba diving to
being a mariner.

This was because in all three cases during my childhood when I was convinced that I would die, I accepted that I would die and in so doing I discovered a wonderful power and that was to extinguish any fear of death and once the fear of death is overcome there really is nothing else that holds any reason to be fearful.

The removal of fear is the greatest of freedoms.

Fear of death is overcome by loving life and by understanding that we are part of a continuum. We are born, we live and we die. This is the natural course of our lives and death is both necessary and inevitable. It is necessary so that new life may emerge. Death is renewal.

I love life. I love being alive and never once during my life have I ever felt depressed or unhappy with being alive. This attitude has made me prepared for the possibility that I could die at any time and being prepared allows for acceptance.

In July 1979, I set out with a ship and a crew of twenty including myself to hunt down the pirate whaler *Sierra*.

I found the ship some 200 miles off the coast of Portugal but due to rough seas I did not take immediate action out of concern for the safety of the crew on the *Sierra*. I needed to control the confrontation.

For that reason, I chased the *Sierra* all the way to the Northern Portuguese port of Leixões, I brought the ship alongside the dock and cleared immigration. The *Sierra* was drifting in the harbor.

When it appeared that the whalers were preparing to take the ship back to sea, I requested clearance from the port authorities. My request was refused. The authorities were intent on helping the *Sierra* escape.

I immediately called a crew meeting and informed everyone that we were going to depart without permission and my intention was to deliberately ram and disable the whaling ship. I told them that most likely they would be arrested so if they did not want to participate, they were free to leave but they had only 10 minutes to do so. Of the nineteen crew, only two men made the choice to stay. Fortunately, they were my engineers. The others stayed on the dock.

We got underway and picked up speed as we moved across the harbor towards the *Sierra*. I gave them a warning blow by striking their harpoon followed by circling around them to hit them at an angle on their port side, splitting their hull open to the water line.

I then headed out to sea but we were stopped by the Portuguese Navy and escorted back to the harbor.

I was taken to the Port captain who said that I should be charged with negligence for ramming the *Sierra*. I responded that there was absolutely nothing negligent about the action. I hit the ship deliberately with the intent to destroy it.

He laughed and said that he could not charge me until he found out who actually owned the whaling ship and said that I was free to go.

After leaving I met up with the crew at a local tavern. One of my crew said to me, "if I knew you were going to get away with it, I would have been there with you."

I smiled and said to him, "sometimes you have to go into a situation where the only thing you can do is to carry out the action."

Weren't you worried about being arrested and sent to prison? Another crewmember asked.

"No. I crossed the ocean for a reason and my objective was to stop that killing machine, no matter the risks. The risks were acceptable."

"But you all could have been killed," said another crewmember.

"Perhaps, but here we are."

Fear is a poison that seeps into the soul and paralyzes our senses generating paranoia, insecurity and anger. Never let fear enter your life.

There is really nothing to fear because things are what they are and will be what they will be. Remember you are the captain of your fate and the master of your soul and body. Who you are and what you wish to be depends on you and you alone. A person free of fear can accomplish far more than a person shackled to fear.

Some Quotes on Fear

> "Fear is the main source of superstition, and one of the main sources of cruelty. To conquer fear is the beginning of wisdom."
> **— Bertrand Russell**

"Fear defeats more people than any other one thing in the world."
— Ralph Waldo Emerson

"I have learned over the years that when one's mind is made up, this diminishes fear; knowing what must be done does away with fear."
— Rosa Parks

Fear is the mind-killer. Fear is the little-death that brings total obliteration. I will face my fear. I will permit it to pass over me and through me.
— Frank Herbert (Dune)

DETACHMENT FROM MATERIALS

Nothing material is permanent and thus objects are not worth stressing about. Your car is damaged, something you own is stolen, or you lost your investments etc. It is really not important. Material objects and comforts are nice but they should not be anchors keeping you attached to stress. Move on.

In December 1979 I had to scuttle my first ship the *Sea Shepherd*. Six months previous I had hunted down, rammed and disabled the pirate whaler *Sierra* in a northern Portuguese port. As a result, my ship was arrested and a judge ordered my ship to be turned over to the company that owned the *Sierra* without a trial or a hearing. My agent told me that the judge had taken a bribe.

I was not going to turn my ship over to a whaling company so on the night of December 31st, 1979 as the town of Leixões was celebrating the New Year, my Chief Engineer Peter Woof and myself quietly boarded the *Sea Shepherd* where it was docked. We opened up the salt water cooling system, flooded the engine room and scuttled the ship.

We left the country the next morning. The whaler *Sierra* had been repaired at great expense and was being ready to return to sea and their illegal whaling operations. They never did. On February 6th, 1980 we blew the bottom out of the ship, and sank it.

The campaign was a success. I had lost my ship but it was the only decision that I could have made. I did not stress about it. We traded a ship

for a ship and our reward was the end
of the bloody career of the most
notorious pirate whaler on the planet.

Within a year, I had raised the funds
to purchase and outfit the *Sea
Shepherd II* in Scotland and we made
plans for the long voyage to Siberia to
document illegal Soviet whaling
operations.

Over the last four decades, I have lost
a few ships. I have had no regrets.
The ships were simply tools to save
lives.

There is a wonderful freedom in non-
attachment to materials. I have never
been one to own things or more
importantly to be owned by material
things. The meaning of the word
"mortgage" comes from the Latin
word "mortis" and the "French
"mort". It evolved into the French

legal term "mortgage" which literally means a death pledge or a death contract.

Mortgages have been a major cause of stress for millions of people. I have always refused to be bound by any death pledge.

Material things be they cars, ships, companies, houses, clothing, art, tools, etc., should never be a cause for stress. It's simply not worth it.

The most important thing in life is your health and the health of your family and the ones you love. Paying attention to your children is much more important than spending time engaged with material pursuits that become a cause for alienation from your family or your own body.

Worrying about such things leads to stress and that diminishes your most valuable asset – your health.

FRIENDS

Friends are friends or they are not.

A true friend will never betray you
and if a "friend" does betray you than
he/she is simply not a friend.

Always walk away from betrayal and
do not stress about it.

True and loyal friends are rare
treasures and should be treated as
such. Loyalty returns loyalty.
Compassion returns compassion.
Courage returns courage. You control
only your own loyalty, compassion
and courage, not that of others. And if
people prove disloyal or they betray
you, the treasure is no longer a
treasure but merely a bauble to be
tossed aside. Never stress about
betrayal or loss. It is what it is.

Over the years I have found only a small handful of people that I can without hesitation call my friends, including an even smaller number that I would regard as lifelong friends.

What set them apart was that they have been friends no matter what. This means loyalty, support and a shared understanding of values. These things create a bond that is strong and interdependent.

I have had all sorts of "friends," that is people that I viewed as friends until they revealed that they were something else. A true friend wants nothing from you except for your friendship and will never allow jealousy, envy, anger, avarice or another person to damage or betray the relationship.

A true friend can't betray you and you can't betray a true friend because the very act of betrayal demonstrates that there never was a true friendship.

I have also found that shared dangerous experiences lead to the most powerful friendships. People who fought in wars together, or climbed mountains and took on challenging explorations. In my case my closest longtime friends shared in the most challenging and riskiest campaigns with me. These experiences create a bond.

Sometimes a person that you felt certain is a friend can betray you. This has occurred with me a couple of times. My position on this has been to never tolerate a betrayal. Experience has taught me that second chances rarely work and it simply is not worth it to stress over any betrayal.

I have had many betrayals, but not by true friends. Those betrayals are easily dismissed. I have no tolerance for betrayal and there can be no second chances.

In the few cases where I felt that someone I considered a true friend betrayed me, I had to accept the situation and acceptance negates stress. This is followed by a rational decision to have nothing to do with the person again.

Friends can disappoint and sometimes they can make you angry and that is forgivable. Betrayal is never forgivable. There is no stress in making decisions based on your boundaries and values.

LONELINESS

Loneliness is an opportunity. It is an opportunity to discover yourself. You can't find someone to love you, if you don't love yourself, and the secret to finding the right person is to not look for that person. Love should blossom from the ground like a lovely wild flower. It cannot be cultivated until after it is realized. Do not seek the seed but let the flower reveal an opportunity to you to grow and learn.

Currently in response to the Covid-19 virus, the policy in most nations is to have people self-isolate. Many people will be placed in a position, where they will be alone and feeling lonely.

In this day and age however, this is not that difficult. We have the advantage of technology and social networks. We can still communicate.

The virus is a very serious threat to the homeless but for those with homes, it should not be that difficult to self-isolate.

If there is a choice between being isolated or contracting the disease, it makes sense to self-isolate. We also need to remember that in addition to the possibility of getting the disease there is also the possibility of passing it on to people whose immune systems can't cope with the virus.

These decisions should be made calmly, rationally and not influenced by worry, fear or stress.

RELATIONSHIPS

Relationships are like streams, constantly flowing and as they flow they meet obstacles. Some are minor and others major but a relationship either flows around the obstacle or it is blocked, and if permanently blocked, it ends. This is not cause for stress or angry resentment or jealously. It is what it is. Move on with appreciation and without bitterness for the relationship that is no more and open your heart to other possibilities that life presents.

The most important factor in maintaining a meaningful relationship with lovers, family or friends is simply acceptance. You need to accept them for who they are and they need to accept you for who you are. If you cannot accept another person for who they are, you need to stop inflicting stress on that person and to walk away. And if another person does not accept you for who you are, you need to walk away no matter the nature of the relationship.

Stress kills and living with a person who does not accept you for who you are, is like living with a person who is slowly killing you.

Life goes on. It may be sad to break up a relationship. There may be feelings of rejection, of jealousy, of anger.

When I look back at relationships where I was rejected or where I made the decision to end a relationship, I have always found that what seemed so important and intense at the time no longer seems to be so important or intense. It was what it was and it is what it is.

People should not stay in an abusive
relationship for any reason and they
should not stress about it. Yes, it takes
courage to walk away some times but
most importantly it takes self-esteem.
No one deserves to be abused or
disrespected and the only remedy for
such things is to move on and not to
be fettered by fear of being alone or
fear of the unknown.

One of the most liberating feelings
one can have is to be secure about
being insecure. This means feeling
comfortable without material,
physical or emotional security.

Relationships should not be co-
dependent. Such relationships are
shallow and constantly stressful. The
solution is to gather the strength to
walk away.

If former lovers respond with acceptance, you can be friends but if not, they should be dismissed. It is not worth the stress of continuing with the insecurities of something that is of no benefit to either person.

I am a tolerant person but I have learned that tolerance has its limitations and at a certain point if the relationship becomes stressful, it needs to be ended permanently.

GOSSIP, RUMORS AND
ACCUSATIONS

Oscar Wilde once said that the only thing worse than being talked about was not being talked about.

People talk, they gossip, they make false accusations, some enjoy insulting and belittling others. They are easily dealt with by ignoring them. Responding to them is what they want, so don't respond. Reacting to them is what they want, so don't react. Such people are not worthy of causing stress to you. They come from a place of insecurity, jealously and fear. It is their stress, and their stress is their problem. It should not be yours.

On Facebook, I found early on that whenever I posted anything, I was assaulted by vicious attacks from people I did not know. Their accusations, criticisms and viciousness meant nothing to me. I did not know them. However. I found that their rants irritated other people and injected a great deal of nastiness and negativity.

The solution was simple. I created a cyber dungeon and tossed them all into it. I have about 10,000 in that dungeon today. I blocked, deleted and banned them, never to hear anything from them again.

As a result, I restored peace and positivity to my social pages.

You should never stress about what anyone says to, or about you. What people think about you is irrelevant because no matter what you do there will be critics.

Years ago, I came across this quote by President Theodore Roosevelt:

"It is not the critic who counts; not the man who points out how the strong man stumbles, or where the doer of deeds could have done them better. The credit belongs to the man who is actually in the arena, whose face is marred by dust and sweat and blood; who strives valiantly; who errs, who comes short again and again, because there is no effort without error and shortcoming; but who does actually strive to do the deeds; who knows great enthusiasms, the great devotions; who spends himself in a worthy cause; who at the best knows in the end the triumph of high achievement, and who at the worst, if he fails, at least fails while daring greatly, so that his place shall never be with those cold and timid souls who neither know victory nor defeat."

Self-confidence negates stress. What anyone says about you is unimportant. There are exceptions. It's always nice to listen to constructive criticism from friends and family. However even so if that criticism is vindictive or motivated by their jealousy, their anger or their judgmental attitudes, feel free to ignore them.

HOKA HEY

Hoka Hey.

It's a good day to die.

It's a Lakota saying and it means to
not fear death and to stand firm for
what you believe in, to fight against
all odds and to never surrender. The
one absolute of life is death. We all
will die. What matters is not dying,
but living. It is how you live that is
important and the only thing
important about dying is how you die.
It should be a death without fear, with
dignity and with acceptance that it is
what it is. The person without fear
dies but once, the person shackled by
fear dies slowly from stress and
anxiety. Accept the inevitable,
embrace the final reality of life and
smile in the face of the infinite. The
real secret to happiness is to not fear

your own death, to not fear failure or ridicule, and not to fear others.

Stress is an obstacle to mindfulness and an impediment to impeccability. Stress is the cause of migraines, cancer and many other ailments. It is the reason people smoke, take drugs, and drink excessively. When people ask me why I've never smoked anything, the reason being is that I have never felt inclined to do so. It never seemed healthy to me and I have always been mindful of the consequences. I think that stress blocks mindfulness of consequences. The same holds true to getting drunk or stoned. Without stress there is no need, nor a desire to do either.

Mindfulness is simply awareness of who you are and what you are doing. A person who is mindful is a person free of stress.

Unfulfilled desire leads to stress. Wanting nothing allows you to appreciate what you have. When you want nothing, you want for nothing. We all have basic needs for food, for warmth and shelter, for clothing and for companionship. Mindfulness allows you to be secure with your basic needs. Everything else is a luxury and although luxuries may be appreciated, you should not depend upon them. Depending upon luxuries leads to stress.

I have never worked a day in my life for the sole purpose of making money. I have never wanted to own anything and although I now do own property and material things, I do not allow those things to own me. I never engage in arguments about money or debts. I tend to avoid debts but when debts occur my position is that they are what they are and certainly not anything to be troubled with.

As far as basic needs, I learned to address this as a teenager when I left home at 15. I had no money, no place to stay, no prospects. I jumped a freight train, rode in the automobiles being transported from Toronto all the way to Vancouver. I arrived and camped in the abandoned gun towers on Wreck Beach and the first thing I did was to go to Vancouver City College to enroll. I found a job, moved out of the gun tower into a single room I rented and went from there. Looking back, I see it as an adventure. I had nothing, but there was no stress. I simply replaced the insecurity of my position into an adventurous experience. I treated every job as a learning experience and working as a longshoreman, teamster, tree planter, warehouse man, short order cook, baker, painter, carpet layer, postman, tour guide, landscaper, and seaman – all were educational experiences.

The truth is that all of life is an adventure, the good and the bad, the ups and the downs, the experiences, the hardships, the thrills and the times that were lonely, happy or difficult. Even the loss of friends and family is simply dealt with by acknowledging that death is as it is. It is inevitable and although we may sincerely mourn we can do so without being stressed. This may be difficult to understand but it is indeed quite possible. With the passing of every friend, with the passing of my own wonderful brother I have silently said "Good-bye" with the appreciation of having known them.

I have gone into situations many times where the risks of injury, death or imprisonment were practically a certainty. My approach has always been acceptance. And amazingly I am still alive and still free. When I have had nothing, I have had everything I need, and when I have risked all, I have usually been successful.

One of the things that concerns me is when I read about, or hear of people, especially young people committing suicide because of bullying. I wish that I could talk to such people before they make such a terminal decision. I would tell them to not let the insecurities and fears of others influence them in any way. I would tell them to accept that all the ridicule, insults, bullying and peer pressure is irrelevant and simply unimportant to who they are. If a parent is unaccepting of who you are, you need to say to them that if you are unacceptable to them they have no right to be your parent and you should walk away from them.

Too many people are enslaved to parents, partners and friends who do not accept them. Un-acceptance and bullying are forms of violence and everyone should walk away from violence with dignity. No one should tell you what to believe, how to think, how to dress, how to behave or to dictate your sexual orientation or condemn you for your compassion, your passion, your imagination and your character. You are who you are and that is what it is, and how it should be, and if others do not tolerate who you are, don't give them the satisfaction of destroying you. Simply symbolically spit in their eye, walk away and concentrate on being who you are for the benefit of yourself. And if anyone is inclined to commit suicide my advice is to commit social suicide instead. That is, to drop out of your life as it is and begin another life, in another place with new ideas. Adventure is the antidote for depression. Take a chance, jump into the unknown and you will be amazed at what is awaiting you after you do.

I am not infallible. I have made mistakes in my life, many of them. I have at times in the past responded with anger although never physical and limited to the poison of the pen. I have let some people down, disappointed others and missed opportunities. But the one thing that I have been able to do in my life is to avoid stress.

At 69, I am healthy, happy, optimistic, a father of a three-year old boy and as passionate as I ever have been. Even more so because I have had the grace of experience and the satisfaction of achievement in those areas that I chose to address.

The point of this posting is this: Do not let stress ruin your health, your love or your life. Dread naught and live the adventure, this adventure that is life. It may well be the only life you will ever have. Even if you believe in the afterlife (oh and don't stress about that either) the fact is you will never know for sure, so no sense wasting the unique life that you have.

A stress-free life is not only possible, it's also essential for your health and your happiness.